The Complete Dash Vegan Snacks Recipes for Busy People

Tasty and Affordable Recipes to Enjoy Every Break and Lose Weight

Naomi Hudson

Table of contents

Popcorn

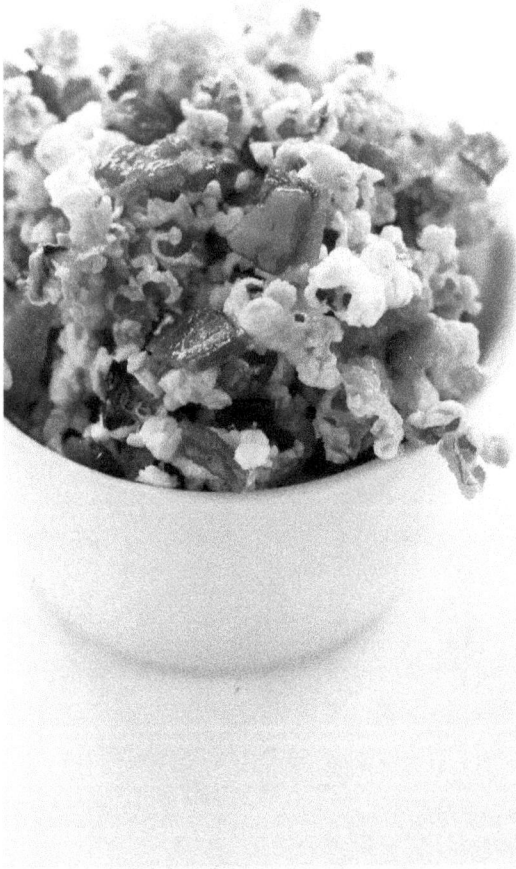

It's a tasty, rather low-calorie snack that can be ready to eat in under 10 minutes. It's perfect if you're craving something a little salty.

Nutritional Facts

servings per container   5

Prep Total   10 min

Serving Size 8

Amount per serving 0%
Calories

% Daily Value

Total Fat 3g   20%

Saturated Fat 4g   32%

Trans Fat 2g 2%

Cholesterol   2%

Sodium 110mg   0.2%

Total Carbohydrate 21g   50%

Dietary Fiber 9g   1%

Total Sugar 1g   1%

Protein 1g

Vitamin C 7mcg   17%

Calcium 60mg   1%

Iron 7mg   10%

Potassium 23mg   21%

Ingredient & Process

1. Place 2 tablespoons of olive oil and ¼ Cup popcorn in a large saucepan.

2. Cover with a lid, and cook the popcorn over a medium flame, ensuring that you are shaking constantly. Just when you think that it's not working, keep on enduring for another minute or two, and the popping will begin.

3. When the popping stops, take off from the heat and place in a large bowl.

4. Add plenty of salt to taste, and if desired, dribble in ¼ Cup to ½ Cup of melted coconut oil. If you are craving sweet popcorn, add some maple syrup to the coconut oil, about ½ Cup, or to taste.

5 Minutes or Less Vegan Snacks

Here's a list of basically 'no-preparation required' vegan snack ideas that you can munch on anytime:

Nutritional Facts

servings per container   5

Prep Total   10 min

Serving Size 8

Amount per serving 0%
Calories

       % Daily Value

Total Fat 20g   190%

Saturated Fat 2g   32%

Trans Fat 1g 2%

Cholesterol   2%

Sodium 70mg   0.2%

Total Carbohydrate 32g   150%

Dietary Fiber 8g   1%

Total Sugar 1g   1%

Protein 3g

Vitamin C 7mcg   17%

Calcium 210mg   1%

Iron 4mg   10%

Potassium 25mg   20%

Ingredients and Process

1. Trail mix: nuts, dried fruit, and vegan chocolate pieces.

2. Fruit pieces with almond butter, peanut butter or vegan chocolate spread

3. Frozen vegan cake, muffin, brownie or slice that you made on the weekend

4. Vegetable sticks (carrots, celery, and cucumber etc.) with a Vegan Dip (homemade or store-bought) such as hummus or beetroot dip. (Careful of the store-bought ingredients though).

5. Smoothie - throw into the blender anything you can find (within limits!) such as soy milk, coconut milk, rice milk, almond milk, soy yogurt, coconut milk yogurt, cinnamon, spices, sea salt, berries, bananas, cacao powder, vegan chocolate, agave nectar, maple syrup, chia seeds, flax seeds, nuts, raisins, sultanas... What you put into your

smoothie is up to you, and you can throw it all together in less than 5 minutes!

6. Crackers with avocado, soy butter, and tomato slices, or hummus spread.

7. Packet chips (don't eat them too often). There are many vegan chip companies that make kale chips, corn chips, potato chips, and vegetable chips, so enjoy a small bowl now and again.

Fresh Fruit

The health benefits of eating fresh fruit daily should not be minimized. So, make sure that you enjoy some in-season fruit as one of your daily vegan snacks.

Nutritional Facts

servings per container   10

Prep Total   10 min

Serving Size 5/5

Amount per serving 1%
Calories

        % Daily Value

Total Fat 24g 2%

Saturated Fat 8g   3%

Trans Fat 4g 2%

Cholesterol   2%

Sodium 10mg   22%

Total Carbohydrate 7g   54%

Dietary Fiber 4g   1%

Total Sugar 1g   1%

Protein 1g   24

Vitamin C 2mcg   17%

Calcium 270mg   15%

Iron 17mg   20%

Potassium 130mg   2%

Ingredients:

1. Chop your favorite fruit and make a fast and easy fruit salad, adding some squeezed orange juice to make a nice juicy dressing.

2. Serve with some soy or coconut milk yogurt or vegan ice-cream if desired, and top with some tasty walnuts or toasted slithered almonds to make it a sustaining snack.

Vegan Brownie

Nutritional Facts

servings per container   3

Prep Total   10 min

Serving Size 7

Amount per serving 20%
Calories

        % Daily Value

Total Fat 3g 22%

Saturated Fat 22g   8%

Trans Fat 17g   21%

Cholesterol   20%

Sodium 120mg   70%

Total Carbohydrate 30g   57%

Dietary Fiber 4g   8%

Total Sugar 10g   8%

Protein 6g

Vitamin C 1mcg   1%

Calcium 20mg   31%

Iron 2mg   12%

Potassium 140mg   92%

Ingredients:

- 1/2 cup non-dairy butter melted

- 5 tablespoons cocoa

- 1 cup granulated sugar

- 3 teaspoons Ener-G egg replacer

- 1/4 cup water

- 1 teaspoon vanilla

- 3/4 cup flour

- 1 teaspoon baking powder

- 1/2 teaspoon salt

1/2 cup walnuts (optional)

Instructions:

1.   Heat oven to 350°. Prepare an 8" x 8" baking pan with butter or canola oil.

2.   Combine butter, cocoa, and sugar in a large bowl.
3.   Mix the egg replacer and water in a blender until frothy.
4.   Add to the butter mixture with vanilla. Add the flour, baking powder, and salt, and mix thoroughly.
5.   Add the walnuts if desired. Pour the batter into the pan, and spread evenly.
6.   Bake for 40 to 45 minutes, or until a toothpick inserted comes out clean.

Spinach Dip

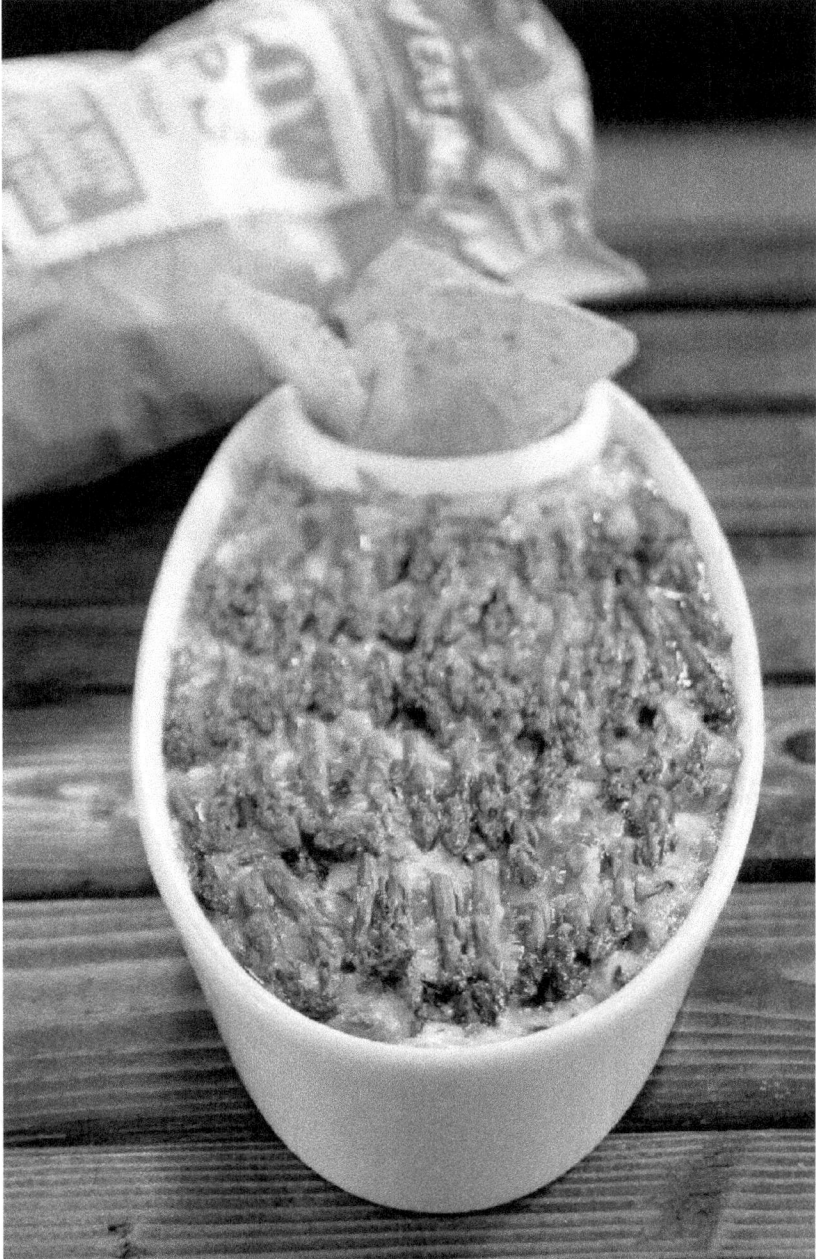

Serving: 2

Prep Time: 4 minutes

Cook Time: 0 minutes

Ingredients:

- 5 ounces Spinach, raw

- 1 cup Greek yogurt

- 1/2 tablespoon onion powder

- 1/4 teaspoon garlic sunflower seeds

- Black pepper to taste

- 1/4 teaspoon Greek Seasoning

How To:

1.   Add the listed ingredients in a blender.

2.   Emulsify.
3.   Season and serve.

Nutrition (Per Serving)

Calories: 101

Fat: 4g

Carbohydrates: 4g

Protein: 10g

Cauliflower Rice

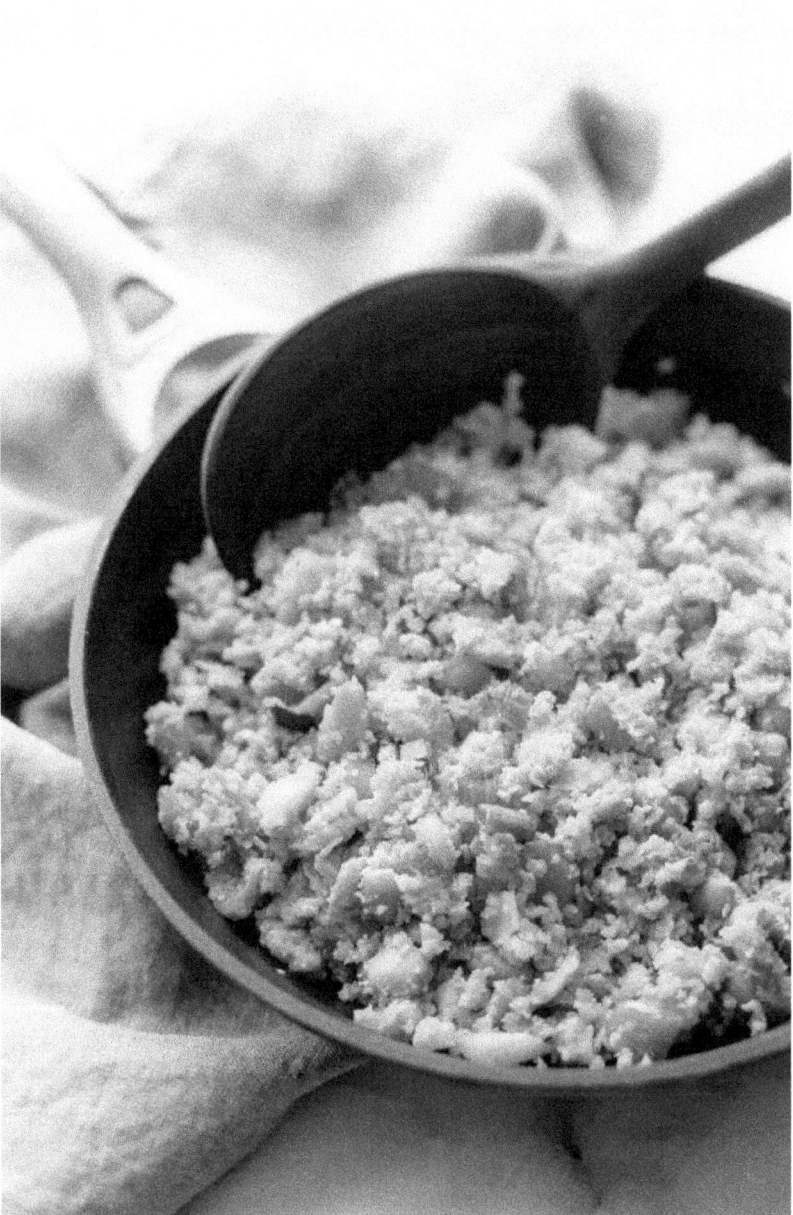

Serving: 2

Prep Time: 5 minutes

Cook Time: 6 minutes

Ingredients:

- 1 head grated cauliflower head

- 1 tablespoon coconut aminos

- 1 pinch of sunflower seeds

- 1 pinch of black pepper

- 1 tablespoon Garlic Powder

- 1 tablespoon Sesame Oil

How To:

1.	Add cauliflower to a food processor and grate it.

2.	Take a pan and add sesame oil, let it heat up over medium heat.

3.	Add grated cauliflower and pour coconut aminos.
4.	Cook for 4-6 minutes.
5.	Season and enjoy!

Nutrition (Per Serving)

Calories: 329

Fat: 28g

Carbohydrates: 13g

Protein: 10g

Grilled Sprouts and Balsamic Glaze

Serving: 2

Prep Time: 10 minutes

Cook Time: 30 minutes

Ingredients:

- ½ pound Brussels sprouts, trimmed and halved Fresh cracked black pepper 1 tablespoon olive oil

- Sunflower seeds to taste

- 2 teaspoons balsamic glaze

- 2 wooden skewers

How To:

1.   Take wooden skewers and place them on a largely sized foil.

2.   Place sprouts on the skewers and drizzle oil, sprinkle sunflower seeds and pepper.
3.   Cover skewers with foil.
4.   Pre-heat your grill to low and place skewers (with foil) in the grill.

5.   Grill for 30 minutes, making sure to turn after every 5-6 minutes.

6.   Once done, uncovered and drizzle balsamic glaze on top.
7.   Enjoy!

Nutrition (Per Serving)

Calories: 440

Fat: 27g

Carbohydrates: 33g

Protein: 26g

Amazing Green Creamy Cabbage

Serving: 4

Prep Time: 10 minutes

Cook Time: 10 minutes

Ingredients:

- 2 ounces almond butter

- 1 ½ pounds green cabbage, shredded

- 1 ¼ cups coconut cream

- Sunflower seeds and pepper to taste

- 8 tablespoons fresh parsley, chopped

How To:

1.   Take a skillet and place it over medium heat, add almond butter and let it melt.

2.   Add cabbage and sauté until brown.
3.   Stir in cream and lower the heat to low.
4.   Let it simmer.
5.   Season with sunflower seeds and pepper.
6.   Garnish with parsley and serve.

7.   Enjoy!

Nutrition (Per Serving)

Calories: 432

Fat: 42g

Carbohydrates: 8g

Protein: 4g

Simple Rice Mushroom Risotto

Serving: 4

Prep Time: 5 minutes

Cook Time: 15 minutes

Ingredients:

- 4 ½ cups cauliflower, riced

- 3 tablespoons coconut oil

- 1-pound Portobello mushrooms, thinly sliced

- 1-pound white mushrooms, thinly sliced

- 2 shallots, diced

- ¼ cup organic vegetable broth

- Sunflower seeds and pepper to taste

- 3 tablespoons chives, chopped

- 4 tablespoons almond butter

- ½ cup kite ricotta/cashew cheese, grated

How To:

1.   Use a food processor and pulse cauliflower florets until riced.

2.   Take a large saucepan and heat up 2 tablespoons oil over medium-high flame.
3.   Add mushrooms and sauté for 3 minutes until mushrooms are tender.
4.   Clear saucepan of mushrooms and liquid and keep them on the side.
5.   Add the rest of the 1 tablespoon oil to skillet.
6.   Toss shallots and cook for 60 seconds.
7.   Add cauliflower rice, stir for 2 minutes until coated with oil.
8.   Add broth to riced cauliflower and stir for 5 minutes.
9.   Remove pot from heat and mix in mushrooms and liquid.
10.   Add chives, almond butter, parmesan cheese.

11.   Season with sunflower seeds and pepper.
12.   Serve and enjoy!

Nutrition (Per Serving)

Calories: 438

Fat: 17g

Carbohydrates: 15g

Protein: 12g

Hearty Green Bean Roast

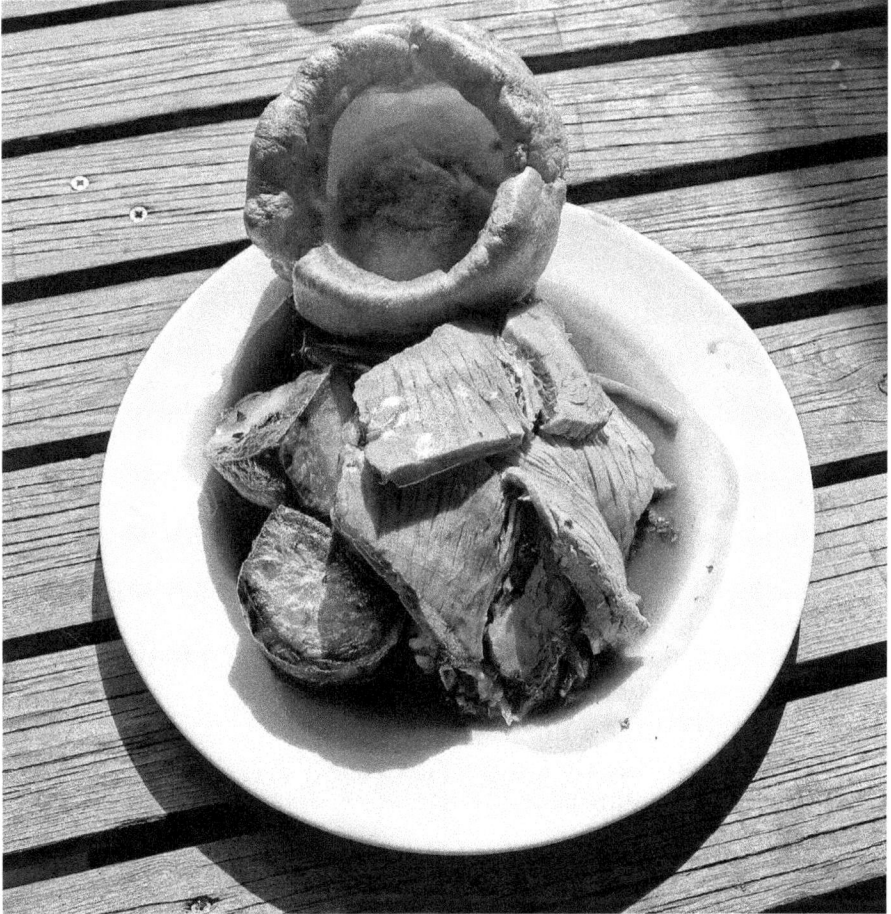

Serving: 4

Prep Time: 10 minutes

Cook Time: 20 minutes

Ingredients:

- 1 whole egg

- 2 tablespoons olive oil

- Sunflower seeds and pepper to taste

- 1-pound fresh green beans

- 5 ½ tablespoons grated parmesan cheese

How To:

1.   Pre-heat your oven to 400 degrees F.

2.   Take a bowl and whisk in eggs with oil and spices.
3.   Add beans and mix well.
4.   Stir in parmesan cheese and pour the mix into baking pan (lined with parchment paper).
5.   Bake for 15-20 minutes.
6.   Serve warm and enjoy!
Nutrition (Per Serving)

Calories: 216

Fat: 21g

Carbohydrates: 7g

Protein: 9g

Almond and Blistered Beans

Serving: 4

Prep Time: 10 minutes

Cook Time: 20 minutes

Ingredients:

- 1-pound fresh green beans, ends trimmed

- 1 ½ tablespoon olive oil

- ¼ teaspoon sunflower seeds

- 1 ½ tablespoons fresh dill, minced

- Juice of 1 lemon

- ¼ cup crushed almonds

- Sunflower seeds as needed

How To:

1.   Pre-heat your oven to 400 degrees F.

2.	Add the green beans with your olive oil and also the sunflower seeds.

3.	Then spread them in one single layer on a large sized sheet pan.

4.	Roast it for 10 minutes and stir, then roast for another 8-10 minutes.

5.	Remove from the oven and keep stirring in the lemon juice alongside the dill.

6.	Top it with crushed almonds and some flaked sunflower seeds and serve.

Nutrition (Per Serving)

Calories: 347

Fat: 16g

Carbohydrates: 6g

Protein: 45g

Tomato Platter

Serving: 8

Prep Time: 10 minutes + Chill time

Cook Time: Nil

Ingredients:

- 1/3 cup olive oil

- 1 teaspoon sunflower seeds

- 2 tablespoons onion, chopped

- ¼ teaspoon pepper

- ½ a garlic, minced

- 1 tablespoon fresh parsley, minced

- 3 large fresh tomatoes, sliced

- 1 teaspoon dried basil

- ¼ cup red wine vinegar

How To:

1.   Take a shallow dish and arrange tomatoes in the dish.

2.   Add the rest of the ingredients in a mason jar, cover the jar and shake it well.
3.   Pour the mix over tomato slices.
4.   Let it chill for 2-3 hours.
5.   Serve!

Nutrition (Per Serving)

Calories: 350

Fat: 28g

Carbohydrates: 10g

Protein: 14g

Lemony Sprouts

Serving: 4

Prep Time: 10 minutes

Cook Time: Nil

Ingredients:

- 1 pound Brussels sprouts, trimmed and shredded

- 8 tablespoons olive oil

- 1 lemon, juice and zested

- Sunflower seeds and pepper to taste

- ¾ cup spicy almond and seed mix

How To:

1.   Take a bowl and mix in lemon juice, sunflower seeds, pepper and olive oil.

2.   Mix well.
3.   Stir in shredded Brussels sprouts and toss.
4.   Let it sit for 10 minutes.
5.   Add nuts and toss.
6.   Serve and enjoy!

Nutrition (Per Serving)

Calories: 382

Fat: 36g

Carbohydrates: 9g

Protein: 7g

Cool Garbanzo and Spinach Beans

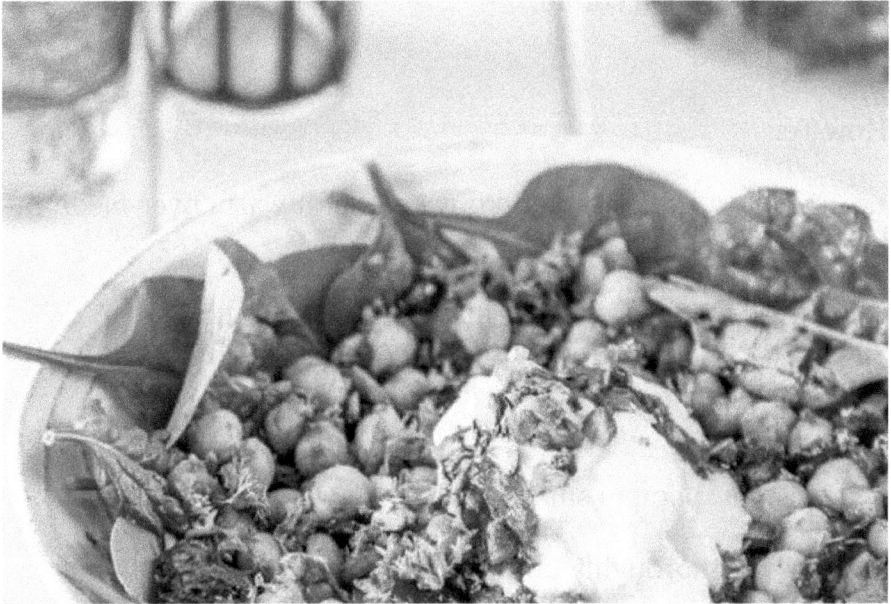

Serving: 4

Prep Time: 5-10 minutes

Cook Time: Nil

Ingredients:

- 1 tablespoon olive oil

- ½ onion, diced

- 10 ounces spinach, chopped

- 12 ounces garbanzo beans

- ½ teaspoon cumin

How To:

1.   Take a skillet and add olive oil, let it warm over medium-low heat.

2.   Add onions, garbanzo and cook for 5 minutes.
3.   Stir in spinach, cumin, garbanzo beans and season with sunflower

seeds.
4.   Use a spoon to smash gently.

5.   Cook thoroughly until heated, enjoy!

Nutrition (Per Serving)

Calories: 90

Fat: 4g

Carbohydrates:11g

Protein:4g

Delicious Garlic Tomatoes

Serving: 4

Prep Time: 10 minutes

Cook Time: 50 minutes

Ingredients:

- 4 garlic cloves, crushed

- 1 pound mixed cherry tomatoes

- 3 thyme sprigs, chopped

- Pinch of sunflower seeds

- Black pepper as needed

- ¼ cup olive oil

How To:

1. Preheat your oven to 325 degrees F.

2. Take a baking dish and add tomatoes, olive oil and thyme.

3. Season with sunflower seeds and pepper and mix.

4.   Bake for 50 minutes.
5.   Divide tomatoes and pan juices and serve.
6.   Enjoy!

Nutrition (Per Serving)

Calories: 100

Fat: 0g

Carbohydrates: 1g

Protein: 6g

Mashed Celeriac

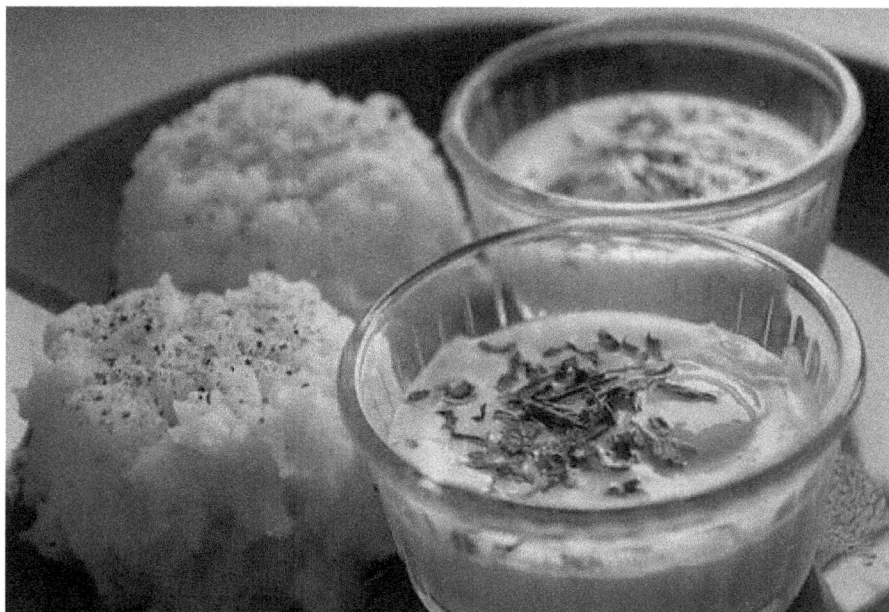

Serving: 4

Prep Time: 10 minutes

Cook Time: 20 minutes

Ingredients:

- 2 celeriac, washed, peeled and diced

- 2 teaspoons extra-virgin olive oil

- 1 tablespoon honey

- ½ teaspoon ground nutmeg

- Sunflower seeds and pepper as needed

How To:

1.   Pre-heat your oven to 400 degrees F.

2.   Line a baking sheet with aluminum foil and keep it on the side.

3.   Take a large bowl and toss celeriac and olive oil.
4.   Spread celeriac evenly on a baking sheet.
5.   Roast for 20 minutes until tender.
6.   Transfer to a large bowl.
7.   Add honey and nutmeg.
8.   Use a potato masher to mash the mixture until fluffy.
9.   Season with sunflower seeds and pepper.
10. Serve and enjoy!

Nutrition (Per Serving)

Calories: 136

Fat: 3g

Carbohydrates: 26g

Protein: 4g

Spicy Wasabi Mayonnaise

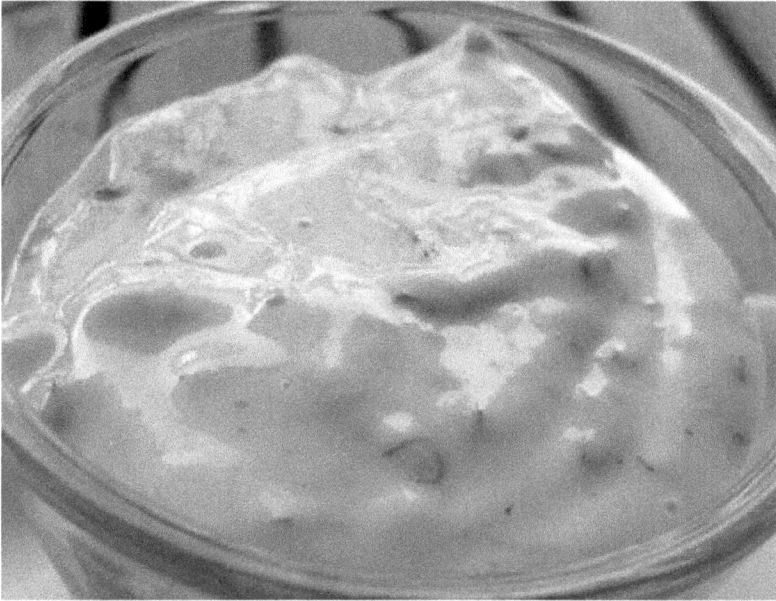

Serving: 4

Prep Time: 15 minutes

Cook Time: Nil

Ingredients:

- 1 cup mayonnaise

- ½ tablespoon wasabi paste

How To:

1.   Take a bowl and mix wasabi paste and mayonnaise.

2. Mix well.
3. Let it chill and use as needed.

Nutrition (Per Serving)

Calories: 388

Fat: 42g

Carbohydrates: 1g

Protein: 1g

Mediterranean Kale Dish

Serving: 6

Prep Time: 15 minutes

Cook Time: 10 minutes

Ingredients:

- 12 cups kale, chopped

- 2 tablespoons lemon juice

- 1 tablespoon olive oil

- 1 teaspoon coconut aminos

- Sunflower seeds and pepper as needed

How To:

1.   Add a steamer insert to your saucepan.

2.   Fill the saucepan with water up to the bottom of the steamer.

3.   Cover and bring water to boil (medium-high heat).

4.   Add kale to the insert and steam for 7-8 minutes.

5.   Take a large bowl and add lemon juice, olive oil, sunflower seeds, coconut aminos, and pepper.
6.   Mix well and add the steamed kale to the bowl.
7.   Toss and serve.
8.   Enjoy!

Nutrition (Per Serving)

Calories: 350

Fat: 17g

Carbohydrates: 41g

Protein: 11g

Spicy Kale Chips

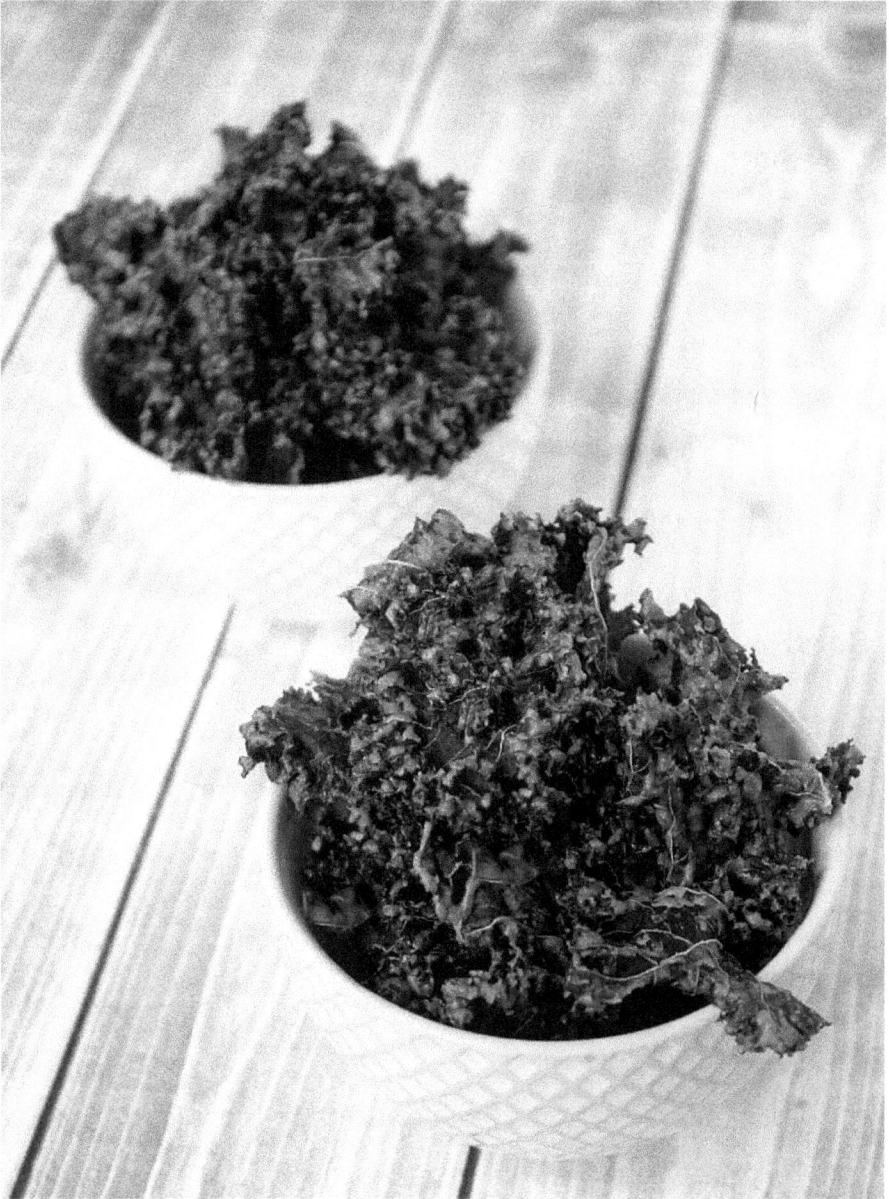

Serving: 4

Prep Time: 10 minutes

Cook Time: 25 minutes

Ingredients:

- 3 cups kale, stemmed and thoroughly washed, torn in 2-inch pieces

- 1 tablespoon extra-virgin olive oil

- ½ teaspoon chili powder

- ¼ teaspoon sea sunflower seeds

How To:

1.   Pre-heat your oven to 300 degrees F.

2.   Line 2 baking sheets with parchment paper and keep it on the side.

3.   Dry kale entirely and transfer to a large bowl.
4.   Add olive oil and toss.
5.   Make sure each leaf is covered.
6.   Season kale with chili powder and sunflower seeds, toss again.

7.   Divide kale between baking sheets and spread into a single layer.

8.   Bake for 25 minutes until crispy.
9.   Cool the chips for 5 minutes and serve.

10. Enjoy!

Nutrition (Per Serving)

Calories: 56

Fat: 4g

Carbohydrates: 5g

Protein: 2g

Seemingly Easy Portobello Mushrooms

Serving: 4

Prep Time: 10 minutes

Cook Time: 10 minutes

Ingredients:

- 12 cherry tomatoes

- 2 ounces scallions

- 4 portabella mushrooms

- 4 ¼ ounces almond butter

- Sunflower seeds and pepper to taste

How To:

1.   Take a large skillet and melt almond butter over medium heat.

2.   Add mushrooms and sauté for 3 minutes.
3.   Stir in cherry tomatoes and scallions.
4.   Sauté for 5 minutes. 5. Season accordingly.
5.   Sauté until veggies are tender.
6.   Enjoy!

Nutrition (Per Serving)

Calories: 154

Fat: 10g

Carbohydrates: 2g

Protein: 7g

The Garbanzo Bean Extravaganza

Serving: 5

Prep Time: 10 minutes

Cook Time: Nil

Ingredients:

- 1 can garbanzo beans, chickpeas

- 1 tablespoon olive oil

- 1 teaspoon sunflower seeds

- 1 teaspoon garlic powder

- ½ teaspoon paprika

How To:

1.   Pre-heat your oven to 375 degrees F.

2.   Line a baking sheet with a silicone baking mat.
3.   Drain and rinse garbanzo beans, pat garbanzo beans dry and put into a large bowl.
4.   Toss with olive oil, sunflower seeds, garlic powder, paprika and mix well.
5.   Spread over a baking sheet.

6.   Bake for 20 minutes.
7.   Turn chickpeas so they are roasted well.
8.   Place back in oven and bake for another 25 minutes at 375 degrees F.
9.   Let them cool and enjoy!

Nutrition (Per Serving)

Calories: 395

Fat: 7g

Carbohydrates: 52g

Protein: 35g

Classic Guacamole

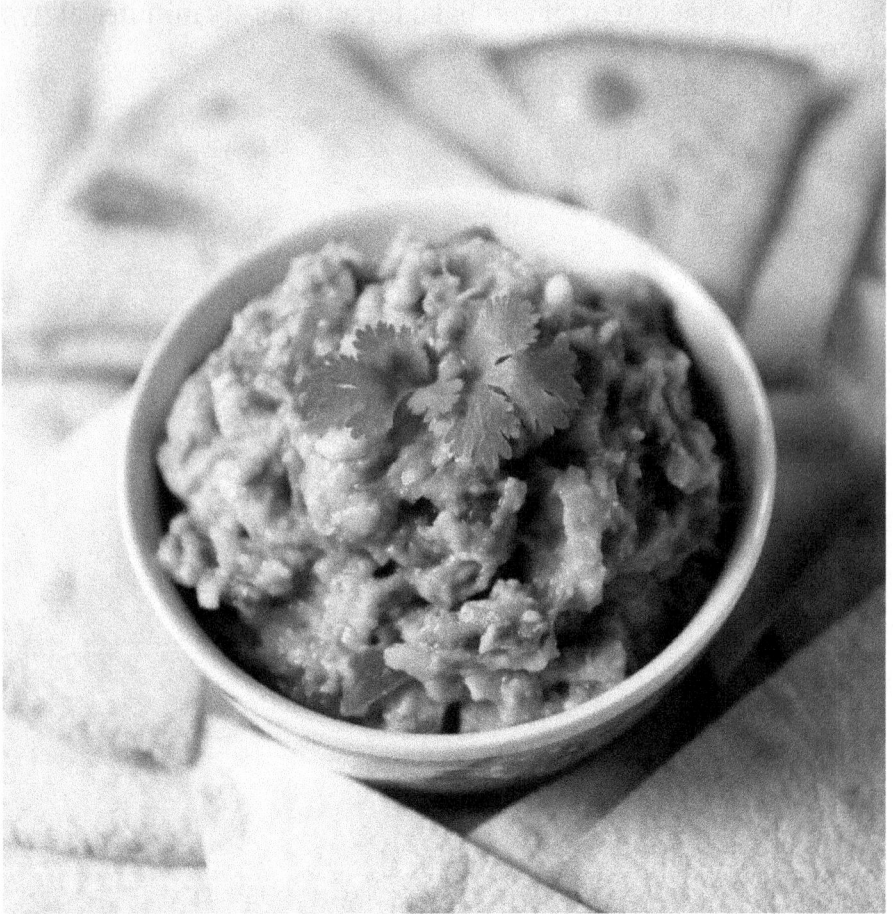

Serving: 6

Prep Time: 15 minutes

Cook Time: Nil

Ingredients:

- 3 large ripe avocados

- 1 large red onion, peeled and diced

- 4 tablespoons freshly squeezed lime juice Sunflower seeds as needed

- Freshly ground black pepper as needed Cayenne pepper as needed

How To:

1. Halve the avocados and discard stone.

2. Scoop flesh from 3 avocado halves and transfer to a large bowl.

3. Mash using a fork.
4. Add 2 tablespoons of lime juice and mix.
5. Dice the remaining avocado flesh (remaining half) and transfer to another bowl.
6. Add remaining juice and toss.
7. Add diced flesh with the mashed flesh and mix.
8. Add chopped onions and toss.
9. Season with sunflower seeds, pepper and cayenne pepper.
10. Serve and enjoy!

Nutrition (Per Serving)

Calories: 172

Fat: 15g

Carbohydrates: 11g

Protein: 2g

Apple Slices

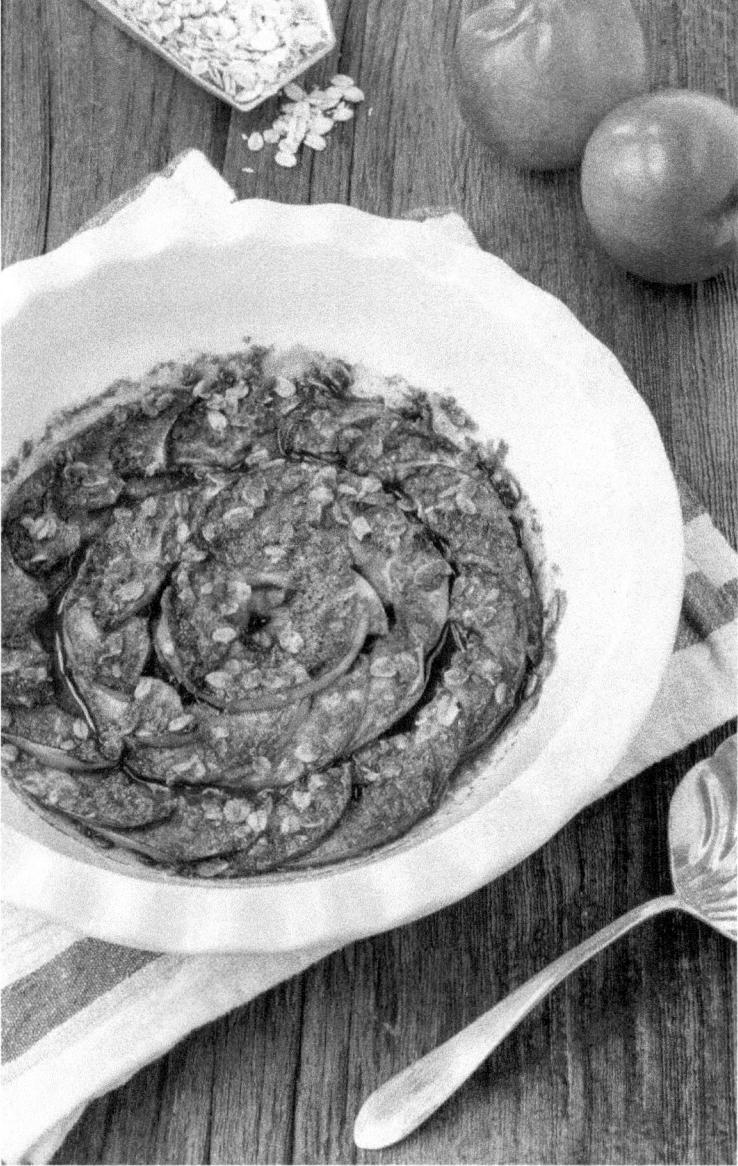

Serving: 4

Prep Time: 10 minutes

Cook Time: 10 minutes

Ingredients:

- 1 cup of coconut oil

- ¼ cup date paste

- 2 tablespoons ground cinnamon

- 4 granny smith apples, peeled and sliced, cored

How To:

1. Take a large sized skillet and place it over medium heat.

2. Add oil and allow the oil to heat up.
3. Stir in cinnamon and date paste into the oil.
4. Add cut up apples and cook for 5-8 minutes until crispy.

5. Serve and enjoy!

Nutrition (Per Serving)

Calories: 368
Fat: 23g

Carbohydrates: 44g

Protein: 1g

Elegant Cashew Sauce

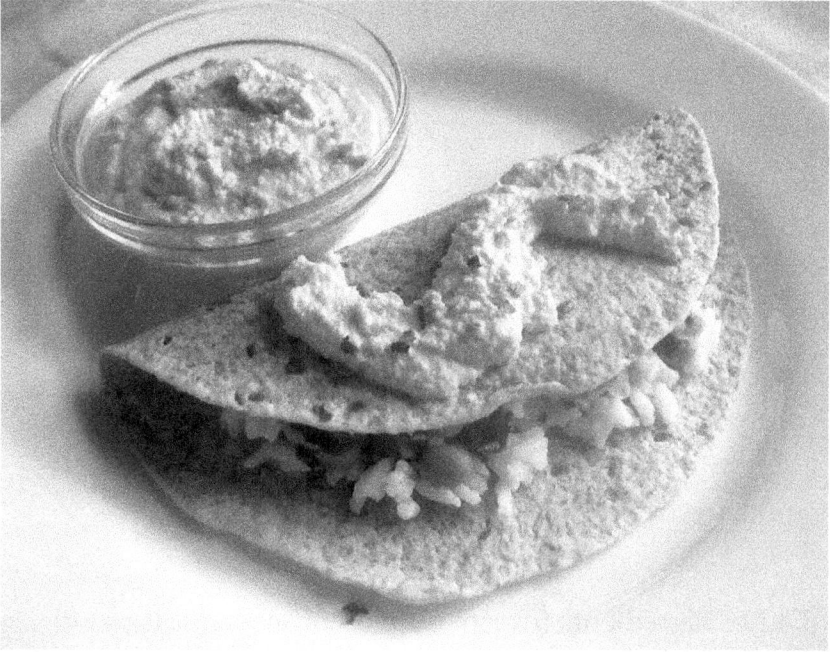

Serving: 4

Prep Time: 5 minutes

Cook Time: Nil

Ingredients:

- 3 ounces cashew nuts

- ¼ cup water

- ½ cup olive oil

- 1 tablespoons lemon juice

- ½ teaspoon onion powder

- ½ teaspoon sunflower seeds

- 1 pinch cayenne pepper

How To:

Add nuts to your blender and process.

Add other ingredients (except oil) and process until smooth .

Add a little bit of oil and puree .

Serve as needed!

Nutrition (Per Serving)

Calories: 361

Fat: 37g

Carbohydrates: 6g

Protein: 3g

Lovely Japanese Cabbage Dish

Serving: 6

Prep Time: 25 minute

Cook Time: Nil

Ingredients:

- 3 tablespoons sesame oil

- 3 tablespoons rice vinegar

- 1 garlic clove, minced

- 1 teaspoon fresh ginger root, grated

- 1 teaspoon sunflower seeds

- 1 teaspoon pepper

- ½ large head cabbage, cored and shredded 1 bunch green onions, thinly sliced 1 cup almond slivers

- ¼ cup toasted sesame seeds

How To:

1.   Add all listed ingredients to a large bowl, making sure to add the wet ingredients first, followed by the dried ingredients.

2.   Toss well to ensure that the cabbages are coated well.
3.   Let it chill and enjoy!

Nutrition (Per Serving)

Calories: 126

Fat: 10g

Carbohydrates: 9g

Protein: 4g

Almond Buttery Green Cabbage

Serving: 4

Prep Time: 10 minutes

Cook Time: 15 minutes

Ingredients:

- 1 ½ pounds shredded green cabbage

- 3 ounces almond butter

- Sunflower seeds and pepper to taste

- 1 dollop, whipped cream

How To:

1.   Take a large skillet and place it over medium heat.

2.   Add almond butter and melt.
3.   Stir in cabbage and sauté for 15 minutes.
4.   Season accordingly.
5.   Serve with a dollop of cream.
6.   Enjoy!

Nutrition (Per Serving)

Calories: 199

Fat: 17g

Carbohydrates: 10g

Protein: 3g

Mesmerizing Brussels and Pistachios

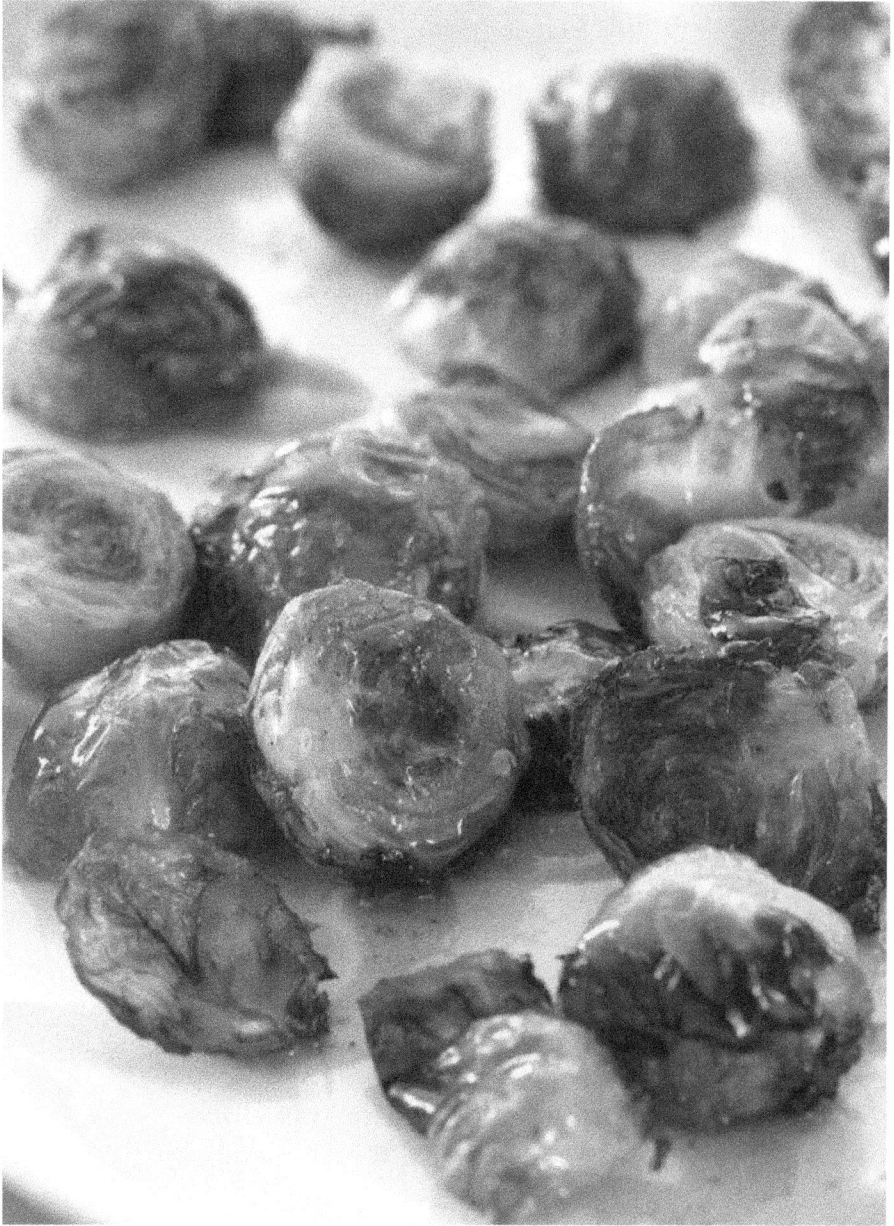

Serving: 4

Prep Time: 15 minutes

Cook Time: 15 minutes

Ingredients:

- 1-pound Brussels sprouts, tough bottom trimmed and halved lengthwise

- 1 tablespoon extra-virgin olive oil

- Sunflower seeds and pepper as needed

- ½ cup roasted pistachios, chopped Juice of ½ lemon

How To:

1. Pre-heat your oven to 400 degrees F.

2. Line a baking sheet with aluminum foil and keep it on the side.

3. Take a large bowl and add Brussels sprouts with olive oil and coat well.
4. Season sea sunflower seeds, pepper, spread veggies evenly on sheet.
5. Bake for 15 minutes until lightly caramelized.
6. Remove from oven and transfer to a serving bowl.
7. Toss with pistachios and lemon juice.
8. Serve warm and enjoy!

Nutrition (Per Serving)

Calories: 126

Fat: 7g

Carbohydrates: 14g

Protein: 6g

Brussels's Fever

Serving: 4

Prep Time: 10 minutes

Cook Time: 20 minutes

Ingredients:

- 2 tablespoons olive oil

- 1 yellow onion, chopped

- 2 pounds Brussels sprouts, trimmed and halved

- 4 cups vegetable stock

- ¼ cup coconut cream

How To:

1.   Take a pot and place it over medium heat.

2.   Add oil and let it heat up.
3.   Add onion and stir-cook for 3 minutes.
4.   Add Brussels sprouts and stir, cook for 2 minutes.
5.   Add stock and black pepper, stir and bring to a simmer.

6.   Cook for 20 minutes more.

7. Use an immersion blender to make the soup creamy.

8. Add coconut cream and stir well.
9. Ladle into soup bowls and serve.
10. Enjoy!
Nutrition (Per Serving)

Calories: 200

Fat: 11g

Carbohydrates: 6g

Protein: 11g

Hearty Garlic and Kale Platter

Serving: 4

Prep Time: 5 minutes

Cook Time: 10 minutes

Ingredients:

- 1 bunch kale

- 2 tablespoons olive oil

- 4 garlic cloves, minced

How To:

1.   Carefully tear the kale into bite sized portions, making sure to remove the stem.

2.   Discard the stems.
3.   Take a large sized pot and place it over medium heat.
4.   Add olive oil and let the oil heat up.
5.   Add garlic and stir for 2 minutes.
6.   Add kale and cook for 5-10 minutes.
7.   Serve!

Nutrition (Per Serving)

Calories: 121

Fat: 8g

Carbohydrates: 5g

Protein: 4g

Acorn Squash with Mango Chutney

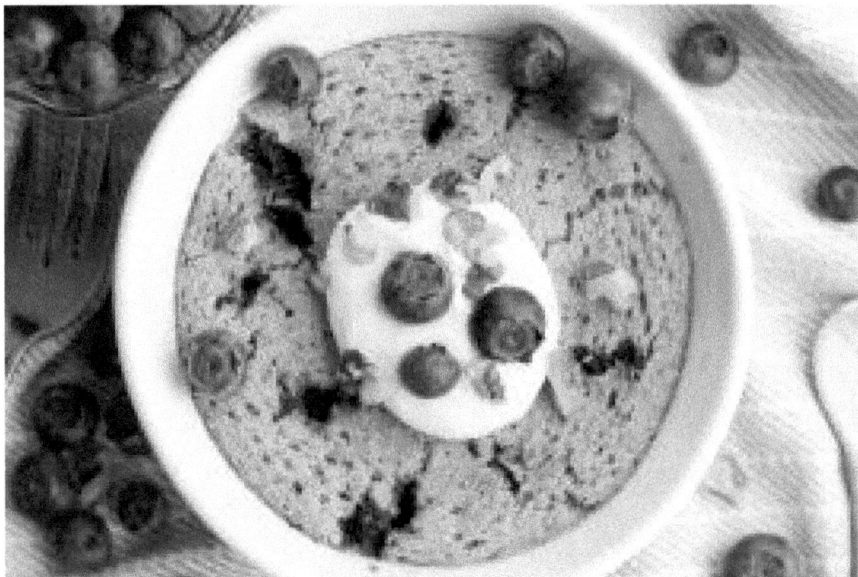

Serving: 4

Prep Time: 10 minutes

Cook Time: 3 hours 10 minutes

Ingredients:

- 1 large acorn squash

- ¼ cup mango chutney

- ¼ cup flaked coconut

- Salt and pepper as needed

How To:

1.   Cut the squash into quarters and remove the seeds, discard the pulp.

2.   Spray your cooker with olive oil.
3.   Transfer the squash to the Slow Cooker and place lid.
4.   Take a bowl and add coconut and chutney, mix well and divide the mixture into the center of the Squash.
5.   Season well.
6.   Place lid on top and cook on LOW for 2-3 hours.

7. Enjoy !
Nutrition (Per Serving)

Calories: 226

Fat: 6g

Carbohydrates: 24g

Protein: 17g

Satisfying Honey and Coconut Porridge

Serving: 8

Prep Time: 10 minutes

Cook Time: 8 hours

Ingredients:

- 4 cups light coconut milk

- 3 cups apple juice

- 2 ¼ cups coconut flour

- 1 teaspoon ground cinnamon

- ¼ cup honey

How To:

1.   In a Slow Cooker, add the coconut milk, apple juice, flour, cinnamon and honey.

2.   Stir well.
3.   Close lid and cook on LOW for 8 hours.
4.   Open lid and stir.
5.   Serve with an additional seasoning of fresh fruits.
6.   Enjoy!

Nutrition (Per Serving)

Calories: 372

Fat: 14g

Carbohydrates: 56g

Protein: 8g

Pure Maple Glazed Carrots

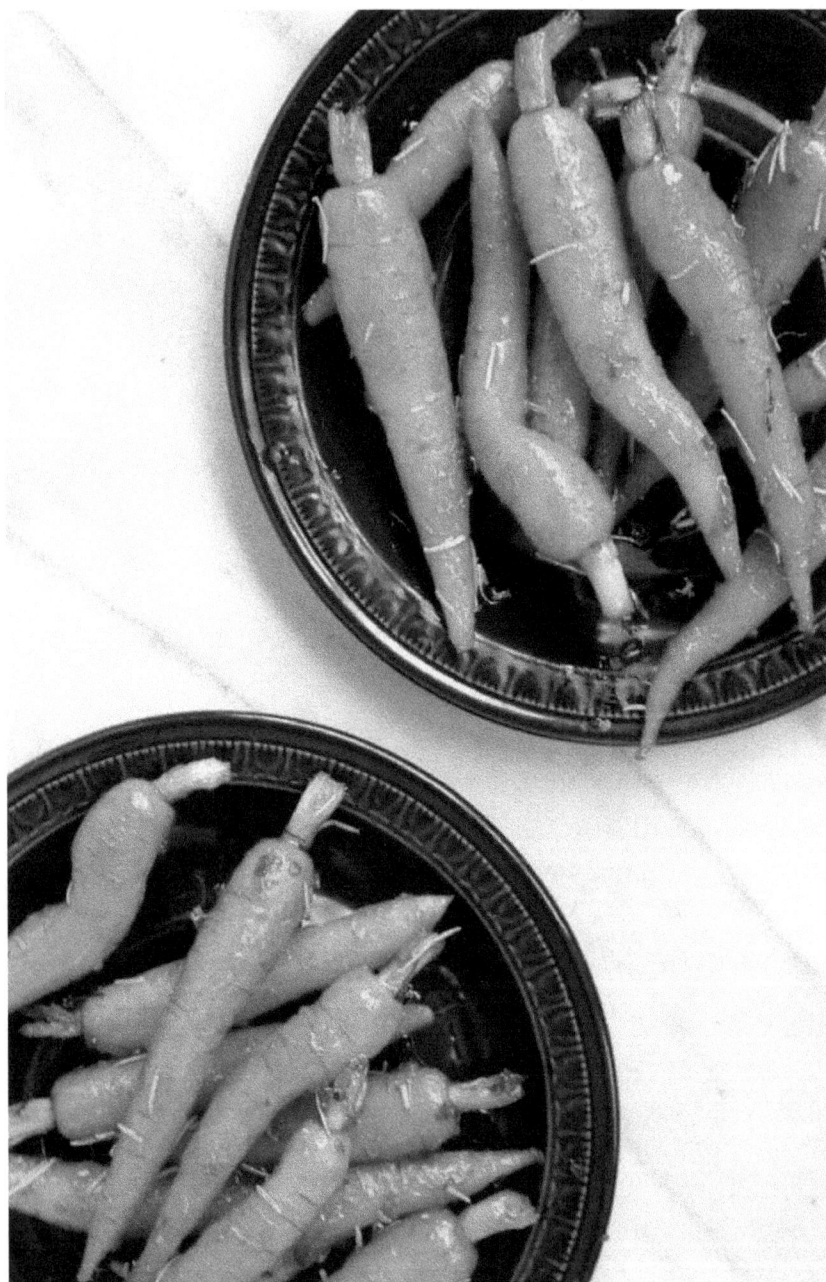

Serving: 6

Prep Time: 10 minutes

Cook Time: 8 hours

Ingredients:

- ¼ cup pure maple syrup

- ½ teaspoon ground ginger

- ¼ teaspoon ground nutmeg

- ½ teaspoon salt

- Juice of 1 orange

- 1-pound baby carrots

How To:

1.   Take a small bowl and whisk in syrup, nutmeg, ginger, salt, orange juice.

2.   Add carrots to your Slow Cooker and pour the maple syrup.
3.   Toss to coat.
4.   Close lid and cook on LOW for 8 hours.
5.   Serve and enjoy!

Nutrition (Per Serving)

Calories: 76

Fat: 1g

Carbohydrates: 19g

Protein: 76g

Ginger and Orange "Beets"

Serving: 6

Prep Time: 20 minutes

Cook Time: 8 hours

Ingredients:

- 2 pounds beets, peeled and cut into wedges

- Juice of 2 oranges

- Zest of 1 orange

- 1 teaspoon fresh ginger, grated

- 1 tablespoon honey

- 1 tablespoon apple cider vinegar

- 1/8 teaspoon fresh ground black pepper Sea salt

How To:

1.   Add beets, zest, orange juice, ginger, honey, pepper, salt and vinegar to your Slow Cooker.

2. Stir well.
3. Close lid and cook on LOW for 8 hours.
4. Serve and enjoy!

Nutrition (Per Serving)

Calories: 108

Fat: 1g

Carbohydrates: 25g

Protein: 3g

Pineapple Rice

Serving: 2

Prep Time: 10 minutes

Cook Time: 2 hours

Ingredients:

- 1 cup rice

- 2 cups water

- 1 small cauliflower, florets separated and chopped ½ small pineapple, peeled and chopped Salt and pepper as needed

- 1 teaspoon olive oil

How To:

1.   Add rice, cauliflower, pineapple, water, oil, salt and pepper to your Slow Cooker.

2.   Gently stir.
3.   Place lid and cook on HIGH for 2 hours.
4.   Fluff the rice with fork and season with more salt and pepper if needed.
5.   Divide between serving platters and enjoy!

Nutrition (Per Serving)

Calories: 152

Fat: 4g

Carbohydrates: 18g

Protein: 4g

Creative Lemon and Broccoli Dish

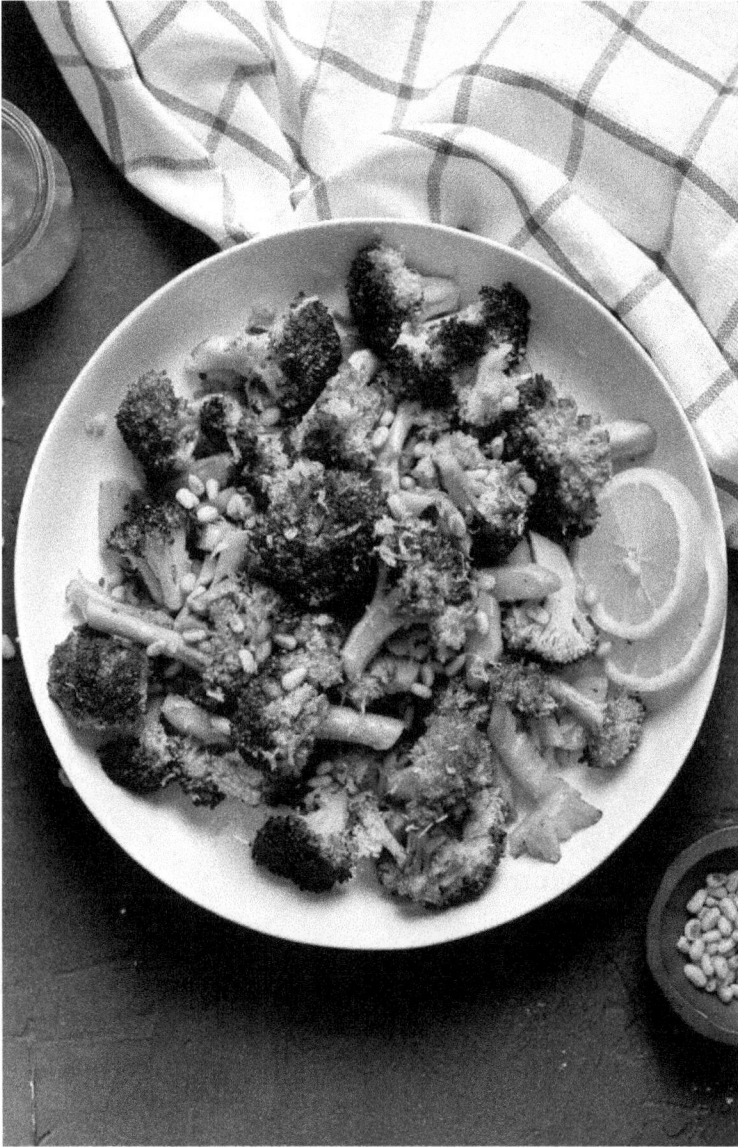

Serving: 6

Prep Time: 10 minutes

Cook Time: 15 minutes

Ingredients:

- 2 heads broccocli, separated into florets

- 2 teaspoons extra virgin olive oil

- 1 teaspoon sunflower seeds

- ½ teaspoon black pepper

- 1 garlic clove, minced

- ½ teaspoon lemon juice

How To:

1. Pre-heat your oven to 400 degrees F.

2. Take a large sized bowl and add broccoli florets.
3. Drizzle olive oil and season with pepper, sunflower seeds and garlic.
4. Spread broccoli out in a single even layer on a baking sheet.
5. Bake for 15-20 minutes until fork tender.
6. Squeeze lemon juice on top.

7. Serve and enjoy!

Nutrition (Per Serving)

Calories: 49

Fat: 1.9g

Carbohydrates: 7g

Protein: 3g

Baby Potatoes

Serving: 4

Prep Time: 10 minutes

Cook Time: 35 minutes

Ingredients:

- 2 pounds new yellow potatoes, scrubbed and cut into wedges

- 2 tablespoons extra virgin olive oil

- 2 teaspoons fresh rosemary, chopped

- 1 teaspoon garlic powder

- ½ teaspoon freshly ground black pepper and sunflower seeds

How To:

1.   Pre-heat your oven to 400 degrees F.

2.   Line a baking sheet with aluminum foil and set it aside.
3.   Take a large bowl and add potatoes, olive oil, garlic, rosemary, sea sunflower seeds and pepper.

4.   Spread potatoes in a single layer on a baking sheet and bake for 35 minutes.
5.   Serve and enjoy!

Nutrition (Per Serving)

Calories: 225

Fat: 7g

Carbohydrates: 37g

Protein: 5g

Cauliflower Cakes

Serving: 4

Prep Time: 10 minutes

Cook Time: 10 minutes

Ingredients:

- 4 cups cauliflowers, cut into florets

- 1 cup kite ricotta/cashew cheese, grated

- 2 eggs, lightly beaten

- 1 teaspoon paprika

- 1 teaspoon chili powder

- Sunflower seeds and pepper to taste

- ½ cup fresh parsley, chopped

- 1 tablespoon olive oil

How To:

1.   Add cauliflower, cheese, paprika, eggs, chili, sunflower seeds, pepper and parsley into a large sized bowl.

2.   Mix well.
3.   Drizzle olive oil into frying pan and place over medium-high heat.

4.   Shape cauliflower mixture into 12 even patties.
5.   Once oil is hot, fry cakes until both sides are golden brown.
6.   Serve hot and enjoy!

Nutrition (Per Serving)

Calories: 180

Fat: 8g

Carbohydrates: 6g

Protein: 8g

Tender Coconut and Cauliflower Rice with Chili

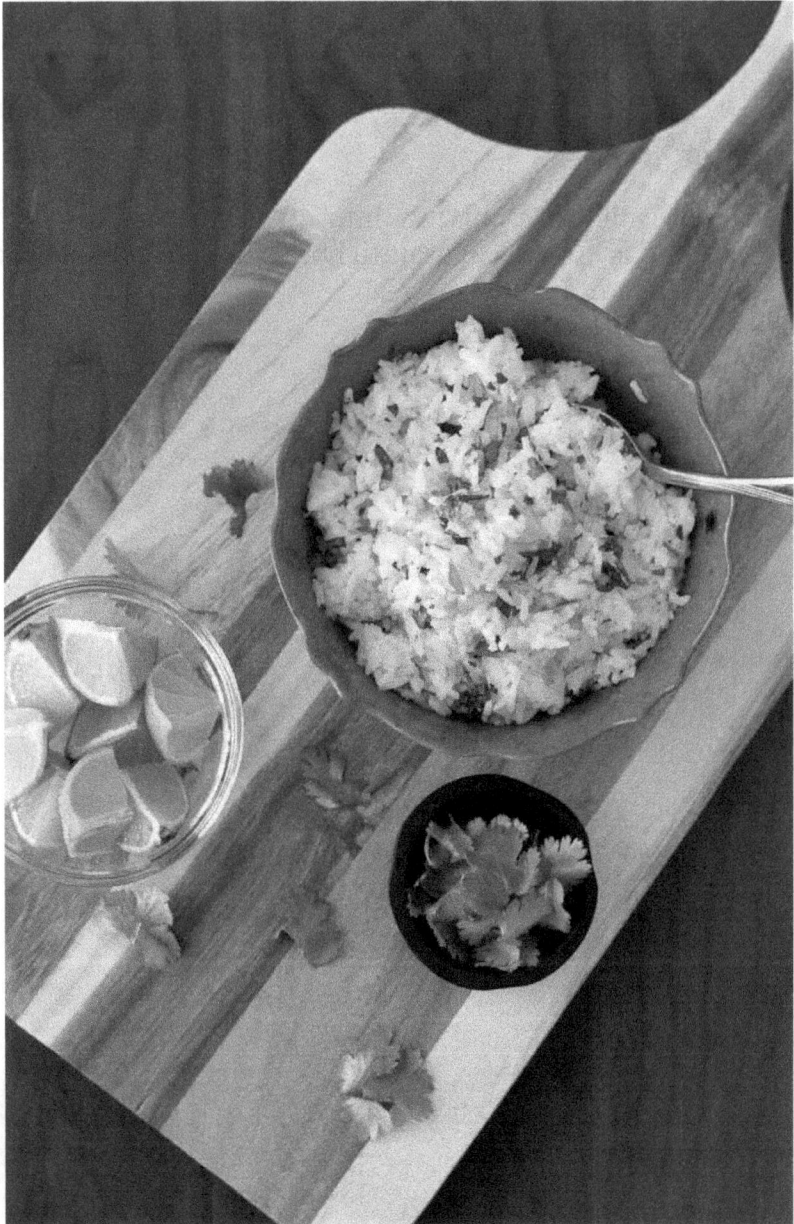

Serving: 4

Prep Time: 20 minutes

Cook Time: 20 minutes

Ingredients:

- 3 cups cauliflower, riced

- 2/3 cups full-fat coconut almond milk

- 1-2 teaspoons sriracha paste

- ¼- ½ teaspoon onion powder

- Sunflower seeds as needed

- Fresh basil for garnish

How To:

1.   Take a pan and place it over medium low heat.

2.   Add all of the ingredients and stir them until fully combined.
3.   Cook for about 5-10 minutes, making sure that the lid is on.
4.   Remove the lid and keep cooking until any excess liquid is absorbed.
5.   Once the rice is soft and creamy, enjoy!

Nutrition (Per Serving)

Calories: 95

Fat: 7g

Carbohydrates: 4g

Protein: 1g

Apple Slices

Serving: 4

Prep Time: 10 minutes

Cook Time: 10 minutes

Ingredients:

- 1 cup of coconut oil

- ¼ cup date paste

- 2 tablespoons ground cinnamon

- 4 Granny Smith apples, peeled and sliced, cored

How To:

1. Take a large sized skillet and place it over medium heat.
2. Add oil and allow the oil to heat up.
3. Stir cinnamon and date paste into the oil.
4. Add sliced apples and cook for 5-8 minutes until crispy.
5. Serve and enjoy!

Nutrition (Per Serving)

Calories: 368

Fat: 23g

Carbohydrates: 44g

Protein: 1g

The Exquisite Spaghetti Squash

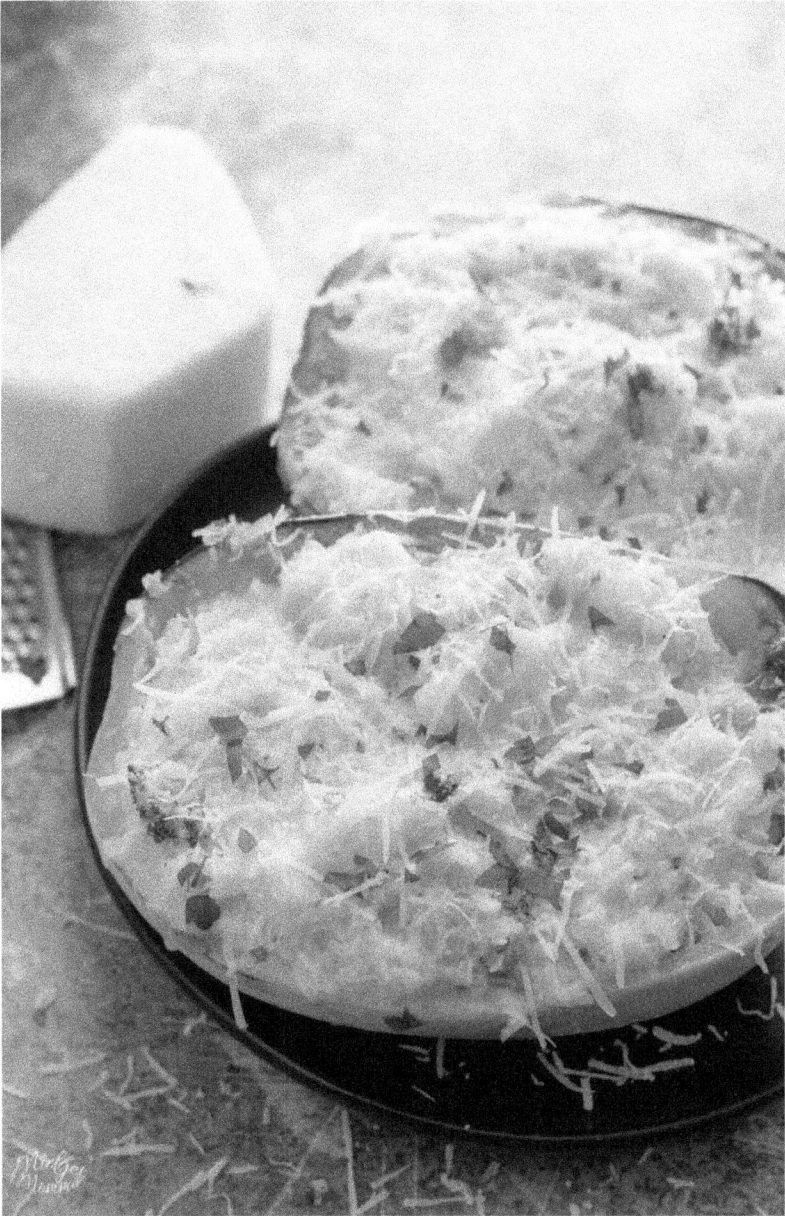

Serving: 6

Prep Time: 5 minutes

Cooking Time: 7-8 hours

Ingredients:

- 1 spaghetti squash

- 2 cups water

How To:

1.   Wash squash carefully with water and rinse it well.

2.   Puncture 5-6 holes in the squash using a fork.
3.   Place squash in Slow Cooker.
4.   Place lid and cook on LOW for 7-8 hours.
5.   Remove squash to cutting board and let it cool.
6.   Cut squash in half and discard seeds.
7.   Use two forks and scrape out squash strands and transfer to bowl.

8.   Serve and enjoy!

Nutrition (Per Serving)

Calories: 52

Fat: 0g

Carbohydrates: 12g

Protein: 1g

The Hearty Garlic and Mushroom Crunch

Serving: 6

Prep Time: 10 minutes

Cooking Time: 8 hours

Ingredients:

- ¼ cup vegetable stock

- 2 tablespoons extra virgin olive oil

- 1 tablespoon Dijon mustard

- 1 teaspoon dried thyme

- 1 teaspoon sea salt

- ½ teaspoon dried rosemary

- ¼ teaspoon fresh ground black pepper

- 2 pounds cremini mushrooms, cleaned

- 6 garlic cloves, minced

- ¼ cup fresh parsley, chopped

How To:

1.   Take a small bowl and whisk in vegetable stock, mustard, olive oil, salt, thyme, pepper and rosemary.

2.   Add mushrooms, garlic and stock mix to your Slow Cooker.
3.   Close lid and cook on LOW for 8 hours.
4.   Open lid and stir in parsley.
5.   Serve and enjoy!

Nutrition (Per Serving)

Calories: 92

Fat: 5g

Carbohydrates: 8g

Protein: 4g

Easy Pepper Jack Cauliflower

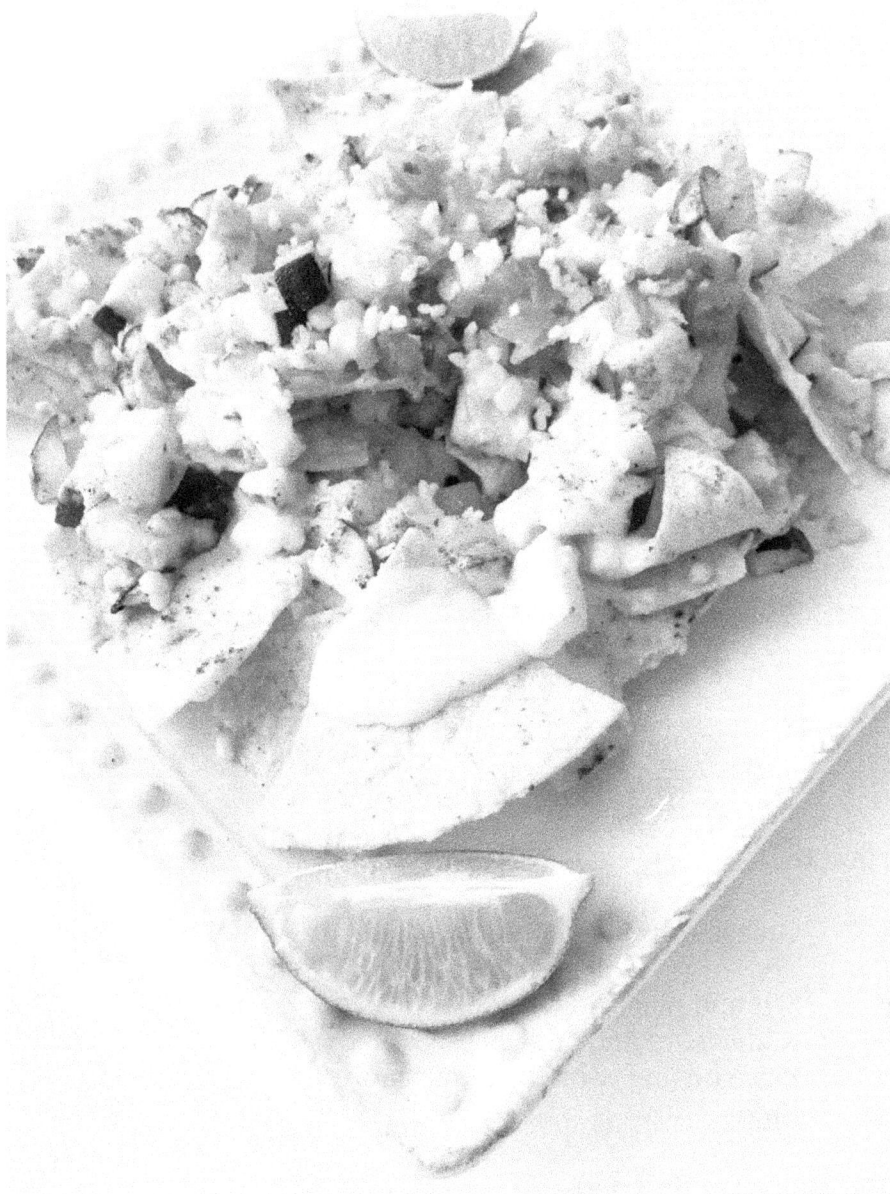

Serving: 6

Prep Time: 10 minutes

Cooking Time: 3 hours 35 minutes

Ingredients:

- 1 head cauliflower

- ¼ cup whipping cream 4 ounces cream cheese

- ½ teaspoon pepper

- 1 teaspoon salt

- 2 tablespoons butter

- 4 ounces pepper jack cheese

How To:

1. Grease slow cooker and add listed ingredients.

2. Stir and place lid, cook on LOW for 3 hours.
3. Remove lid and add cheese, stir.
4. Place lid and cook for 1 hour more.
5. Enjoy!

Nutrition (Per Serving)

Calories: 272

Fat: 21g

Carbohydrates: 5g

Protein: 10g

The Brussels Platter

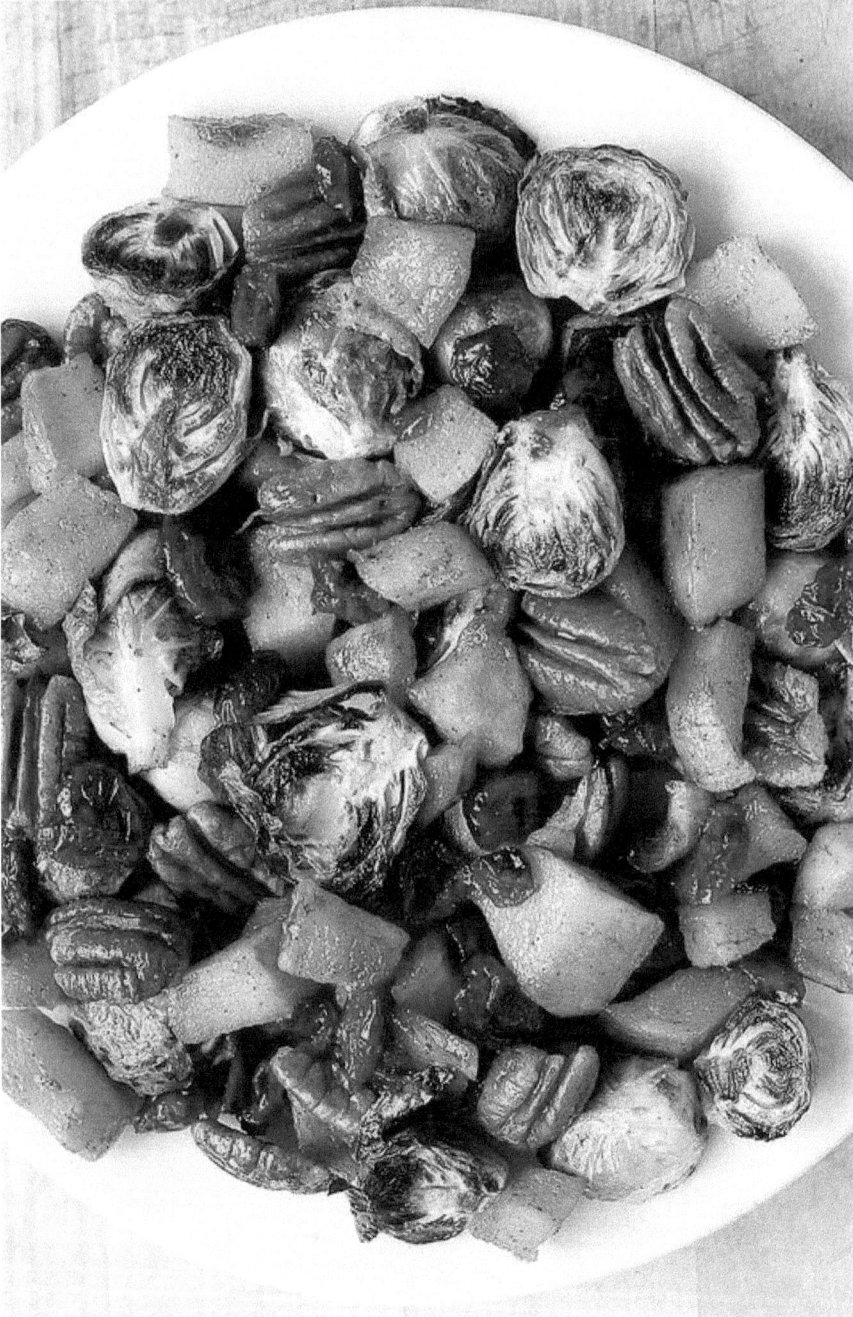

Serving: 4

Prep Time: 15 minutes

Cooking Time: 4 hours

Ingredients:

- 1 pound Brussels sprouts, bottoms trimmed and cut

- 1 tablespoon olive oil

- 1 ½ tablespoons Dijon mustard

- Salt and pepper to taste

- ½ teaspoon dried tarragon

How To:

1.   Add Brussels sprouts, mustard, water, salt and pepper to your Slow Cooker

2.   Add dried tarragon. 3. Stir well and cover.
3.   Cook on LOW for 5 hours, making sure to keep cooking until the Brussels sprouts are tender.
4.   Stir well and arrange.
5.   Add Dijon over the Brussels sprouts.
6.   Enjoy!

Nutrition (Per Serving)

Calories: 83

Fat: 4g

Carbohydrates: 11g

Protein: 4g

The Crazy Southern Salad

Serving: 2

Prep Time: 10 minutes

Cook Time: nil

Ingredients:

- 5 cups Romaine lettuce

- ½ cup sprouted black beans

- 1 cup cherry tomatoes, halved

- 1 avocado, diced

- ¼ cup almonds, chopped

- ½ cup of fresh cilantro

- ½ cup of Salsa Fresca

How To:

1.   Take a large sized bowl and add lettuce, tomatoes, beans, almonds, cilantro, avocado, Salsa Fresco

2. Toss everything well and mix them
3. Divide the salad into serving bowls and serve!
4. Enjoy!

Nutrition (Per Serving)

Calories: 211

Fat: 16g

Carbohydrates: 6g

Protein: 10g

Kale and Carrot with Tahini Dressing

Serving: 1

Prep Time: 15 minutes

Cook Time: nil

Ingredients:

- Handful of kale

- 1 tablespoon tahnini

- ½ head lettuce

- Pinch of garlic powder

- 1 tablespoon olive oil

- Juice of ½ lime

- 1 carrot, grated

How To:

1.   Add kale and roughly chopped lettuce to a bowl.

2.   Add grated carrots to the greens and mix.

3.   Take a small bowl and add the remaining ingredients, mix well.

4.   Pour dressing on top of greens and toss.

5.   Enjoy!

Nutrition (Per Serving)

Calories: 249

Fat: 11g

Carbohydrates: 35g

Protein: 10g

Crispy Kale

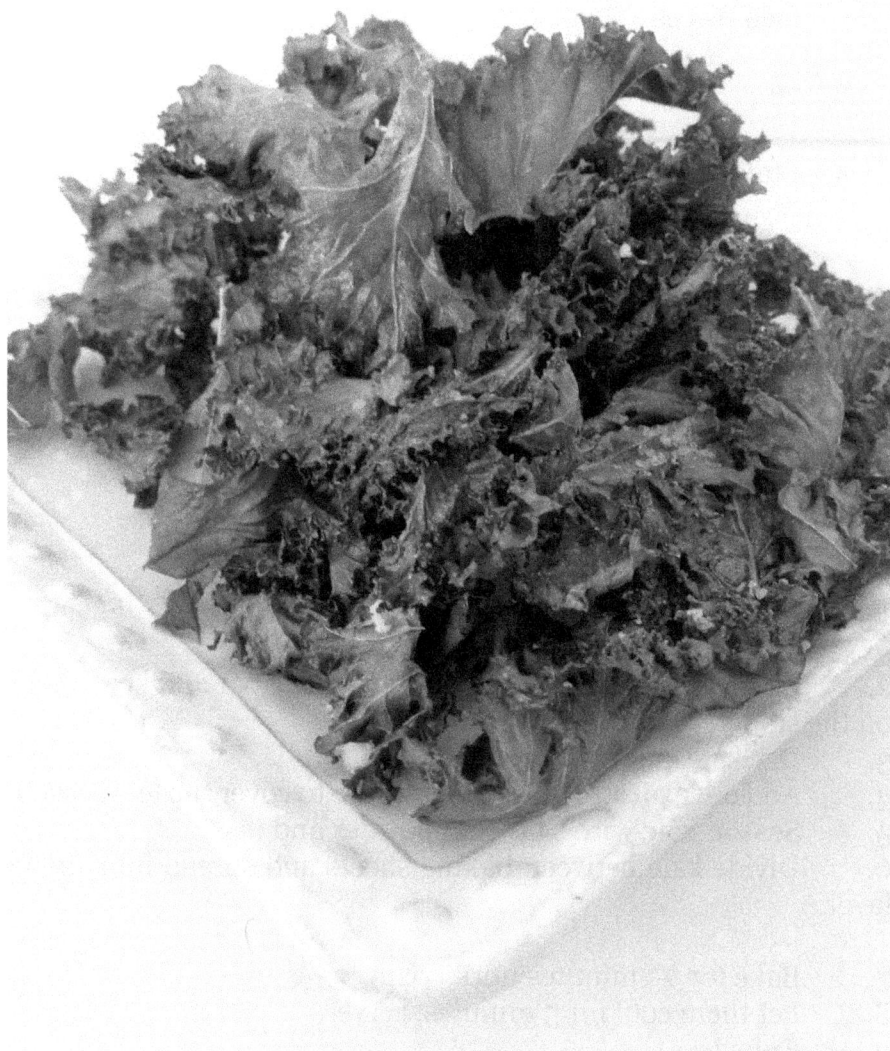

Serving: 4

Prep Time: 10 minutes

Cook Time: 25 minutes

Ingredients:

- 3 cups kale, stemmed and thoroughly washed, torn in 2-inch pieces

- 1 tablespoon extra-virgin olive oil

- ½ teaspoon chili powder

- ¼ teaspoon sea salt

How To:

1. Prepare your oven by pre-heating to 300 degrees F.

2. Line 2 baking sheets with parchment paper and keep them on the side.
3. Dry kale and transfer to a large bowl.
4. Add olive oil and toss, making sure to cover the leaves well.
5. Season kale with salt, chili powder and toss.
6. Divide kale between baking sheets and spread into single layer.

7. Bake for 25 minutes until crispy.
8. Let them cool for 5 minutes, serve.
9. Enjoy!

Nutrition (Per Serving)

Calories: 56

Fat: 4g

Carbohydrates: 5g

Protein: 2g

www.ingramcontent.com/pod-product-compliance
Lightning Source LLC
Chambersburg PA
CBHW050749030426
42336CB00012B/1731